STAYING FIT , SLIMER AND STRONGER.

HIDDEN SECRETS TO BUILDING THE PERFECT BODY.

Matthew Dory Ph.D.

HIDDEN SECRETS TO BUILDING THE PERFECT BODY.

TABLE OF CONTENT

REGULARLY STRETCH WHILE STANDING UP.

EXERCISE RELAXATION TECHNIQUES.

HAVE A RESTFUL NIGHT'S SLEEP.

FREQUENT QUESTIONS I GET ASKED AND MY ANSWERS.

CHAPTER FIVE

YOU CAN EAT EVERYTHING YOU WANT AND STILL LOSE WEIGHT.

CHAPTER SIX

SELECTING MEALS TO REDUCE WEIGHT

CHAPTER SEVEN

HOW TO BREAK AN ADDICTION TO EATING.

CONSIDERATIONS

HOW LONG WILL IT TAKE ME TO GET FIT?

CHAPTER EIGHT

THE MOST COMMON FITNESS MYTHS.

INTRODUCTION

Is this a fitness manual that promises to give you a toned "Hollywood babe figure" in just 30 days?

No.

Does it provide food and workout "hacks" for growing lean muscle and losing belly fat more quickly than a sneeze in a cyclone? Is it a bodybuilding book?

Without a doubt.

But does it provide a detailed guide to eating well, exercising, and losing up to 35 pounds of fat (or more) while building impressive amounts of strength and muscle definition?

Yes.

And more quickly than you likely believe is feasible.

Because of the following:

It's not nearly as difficult to develop muscle and lose fat as you've been made to think.

You are exempt from: Become fixated on eating "clean" and staying away from "bad" things like bread, sweets, and meat. Some meals are healthier than others and need to be consumed more frequently. I'm done now.

You are exempt from: Spend a few hours each day in the gym toiling through taxing strength training routines. For developing lean muscle and strength, sweating profusely, becoming really painful, and working until you are bone-tired are all completely overrated. You're not required to: Work out on the treadmill. In reality, you may construct your finest physique ever and lose unsightly belly, hip, and thigh fat without ever engaging in any physical activity.

These are only a few of the damaging beliefs and lies that prevent women from ever reaching the slim, toned, and powerful figure they genuinely want.

And this book will impart knowledge on you that the majority will never acquire:

How to change your physique while consuming the foods you enjoy and engaging in only a few difficult but manageable resistance training sessions each week. Oh, and exercise? entirely optional.

CHAPTER ONE

WHAT YOU SHOULD KNOW ABOUT LOSING WEIGHT.

3500 calories make up one pound of body weight. This indicates that if your daily calorie consumption is reduced (or increased) by 500, you will lose (or gain) 1 pound a week. (3500 calories) (500 calories each day multiplied by 7 days).

Carbohydrate, protein, and fat are present in all foods. 1 gram of carbohydrates has 4 calories. One gram of protein has 4 calories. Fat offers 9 calories per gram.

Either simple or complex carbohydrates exist. Compared to complex carbs, simple carbohydrates contribute to increased weight gain. Starches and sugar are examples of simple carbohydrates (potatoes, pasta, and rice). Complex carbohydrates include things like fruits, vegetables, and entire grains.

THINGS YOU CAN TAKE TO LOSE WEIGHT.
Understand where you are going. For three to five days, keep a food journal. Eat what you typically eat during this time. Record everything you consume in writing. For foods without a nutrition label, measure servings. Calculate the total number of

calories and the grams of carbohydrate, protein, and fat for each item. (You may find this information via computer programs, smartphone applications, or books that measure calories. You may get a database of food nutrients at ndb.nal.usda.gov/ndb/foods.) Keep track of the total calories and the grams of carbohydrate, protein, and fat for each food.

Identify The Issue, Analyze Your Daily Caloric Intake.
You are consuming too many calories if you are gaining weight. You already know that this number of calories is effective for weight management if your weight is stable. To lose weight, however, you must reduce your calorie consumption.

Fix The Issue.
Eat less of (or stop eating) foods with empty calories. These foods don't supply you with enough of the nutrients you require. Sodas, booze, and sweets are a few examples.

Choose A Sensible Calorie Target.
Start by reducing your daily calorie consumption by 500 to 1000. Within this range, modify your calorie intake to promote weekly weight loss of 1 to 2 pounds. You can cut back even more if you are comfortable after one or two weeks and wish to lose weight more rapidly. Do not, without a doctor's supervision, consume less than 1000 calories each day. Those who consume 3000 calories per day

might lose weight in some cases. Some people might need to keep their daily calorie intake at 1100.

There isn't a perfect ratio of carbs, proteins, and fats for weight loss. However, the majority of health professionals advise eating a balanced diet that contains between 15 and 20 percent of calories from protein, 20 to 35 percent from fat, and the remaining calories from complex carbs.

Be Careful To Get Adequate Protein.
The daily need for a lady of average size is 50–60 grams. A guy of average size need 65 to 75 grams each day. Your requirements for protein may be significantly higher if you are larger, more active, or unwell. If you feel hungry after regular meals, eat additional protein. Your metabolism will slow down if you only have a modest salad throughout the day. If you want to reduce weight, this is not beneficial. Here are some examples of typical protein content in typical foods: Three ounces of lean meat weighs 25 grams, three ounces of fish weighs 20, eight ounces of milk weighs eight, one ounce of cheese weighs seven, and one egg weighs six.

Snack On Fruit And Veggies.
Consider replacing chips with baby carrots or celery sticks with salsa. Instead of chocolate chips, use berries. Apples are preferable than apple pie.

You must alter your behaviors if you want to reduce weight. This will develop gradually. Losing 1 to 2 pounds a week is a significant achievement. Better health and wellbeing should be your main priorities. If you have serious health issues, see a doctor. Type 2 diabetes, heart disease, and renal disease are a few examples of such issues. Consult your doctor if you regularly use drugs since the dosages might need to be changed as you lose weight. In the event that you have diabetes or high blood pressure, this is extremely crucial.

Pick A Pleasant Hobby, Then Get Moving.
Walk or trek, for instance. Attend courses in tap dance or tai chi. or sign up for a basketball or bowling league. Exercise will assist you tone your muscles and prevent sagging skin. Muscle is developed by exercise. You will burn more calories each day as a result. Try to exercise daily for at least 30 minutes. A quick 10-minute stroll offers advantages. To keep track of how far you walk each day, wear a pedometer (step counters). They could even motivate you.

It takes more than simply a healthy diet and exercise to lose weight. There wouldn't be as many diets and methods to choose from if losing weight were simple. Every diet and weight-loss plan has benefits and drawbacks, but for any of them to be effective, you need to have the appropriate mindset.

The key aspect in losing weight, according to New York City-based therapist, is changing your thinking about how to lose weight. Without having the right inner resolve and intention, we cannot transfer our weight from the outside. And the majority of individuals attempt to lose weight while feeling the worst kind of way: that they need to "fix" themselves. When they feel ashamed or disgusted with themselves, they immediately start diets and workout regimens while pinching their "problem" areas, calling themselves "fat," and generally feeling inferior. They get fixated on outcomes, place too much emphasis on short remedies, and overlook sustainability and even health.

According to a North Carolina-based cardiologist, "This kind of thinking might be harmful." "These people concentrate on negative ideas rather than the benefits of losing weight, such as improved health, a longer life, more enjoyment in daily activities, and the avoidance of diabetes and heart disease. Negative thinking ultimately results in failure. According to science, changing your thinking is necessary for diet success.

Yes, changing your mindset regarding weight reduction is about more than simply sentimentality; it's about getting results. In fact, according to Syracuse University studies, women are more prone to forgo exercise the unhappier they are with their bodies. Additionally, a 2015 study that was published in the International Journal of Obesity found that merely believing that you are overweight predicts future weight increase.

Psychologists emphasize that your behaviors are predicted by how you view yourself and your fundamental identity: You will behave as you would if you believed that you were overweight, opposed to exercise, or undeserving. But biology could possibly be involved.

The stress hormone cortisol, which your adrenal glands release whenever you feel sorry on yourself or worry about how you look on the scale, has been proven in several studies to enhance the distribution of fat around the belly.

Thankfully, the mind is a malleable entity. To alter your perspective and make your weight-loss strategy healthier, happier, and more effective, follow these 15 expert-approved ideas.

UNDERSTAND WHY.

According to a licensed naturopath, exercise physiologist, and director of physical activity at Newtopia, a Toronto-based health company focused on chronic disease prevention through sustainable habit change, when attempting to make meaningful and long-lasting changes to habits, including those that you'll need to shift to become successful with dieting, you need to examine your motivation.

Being honest with yourself and understanding that changing your habits will be necessary for success are things Vani advises. Are you prepared to make these adjustments and take the required actions to lose weight in a healthy and lasting way?

Good decisions need preparation, practice, and understanding of barriers in order to do this. One of the primary reasons diets fail is because dieters fall prey to various types of sabotage and get caught in a deadly loop.

Put Education First.
A Breakthrough Solutions' creator and New York City-based certified mental health counselor I know thinks it's "extremely important to understand how different meals effect your body and how different workouts impact your body as well. It is really beneficial to have an attitude of learning about your physical fitness.

developing lasting health habits is a process that involves the full individual and is also impacted by sleep and outside variables like social life and stress.

Practice Making Decisions With Awareness.
knowing the behavioral significance that meals have in our life helps us recognize and practice the choices we make. The short- and long-term success

of diets is determined by these decisions. For instance, mindful eating, also known as intuitive eating, is a method of eating that aims to comprehend your eating habits and feelings. You may develop a conscious link between your thoughts and decisions and the reasons you first go for the unhealthy selections by tracking and monitoring your emotions related to food choices.

Modify your targets.
Although weight loss may be an outcome, it shouldn't be the main objective. a clinical and consultant psychotherapist located in New York City advises setting small, attainable goals that you have complete control over. Did you, for instance, have five servings of fruits and vegetables today? One objective was achieved.

How about a good night's sleep? Have you admitted them? In such case, you may cross another item off your list.

Big goals are fine to have, but achieving them may be daunting, according to chief of psychology at Noom, the well-known behavior modification and weight-loss app and program. Instead, consider breaking your major objective down into more manageable steps.

Making **SMART** objectives is a wise practice:

Specific.
Measurable.
Attainable.
Realistic.
Time-bound.
"If your objective is to wake up early every morning to run but you haven't run in a while, start by just rising earlier or deciding to stroll instead of jogging. Over time, you could increase how much time you devote to working out. Think of each activity as a brick in a structure. Small first steps might result in more significant changes "He asserts.

Tend To Be Optimistic.
I personally suggest surrounding oneself with uplifting people. By doing this, you may make an investment in yourself in a safe, emotionally stable environment. Don't be hesitant to ask for help or guidance, If you have a buddy, partner, or coach at your side, you can maintain accountability.

Obtain Wise Counsel From Reliable People.
This may considerably assist you understand what specifically works best for you, and some solutions are even accessible under your employer's health care plan. Knowing what works for you is crucial since losing weight may be a highly individual process. there is basically no one way to approach asking for help with weight-loss programs that is

appropriate or wrong since everyone has varied criteria to best suit their personal interests.

Online resources, medical guidance, support alternatives through workplace wellness programs, and even instructional books about weight loss and dieting are available to dieters.

Try looking to one of those sources for knowledge and direction if you're having trouble succeeding, or if you're uneasy or feeling discouraged. Additionally, a therapist "can be a confidant, assist address those hurdles that limit growth and discover good strategies to break harmful patterns, if you need to talk about any more profound difficulties, it may be a good idea to get treatment from a mental health professional if you have had "previous experiences with disordered eating, including substantial anxiety surrounding eating or bad exercise routines." A mental health expert may also be able to assist you if you're having trouble with your "body image, feel compelled to lose weight but don't completely understand why, or simply need a sounding board as you try to navigate making this change." We have discovered that asking for help frequently and early boosts the chance of success. Rethink the use of rewards and penalties. As a certified dietitian, author, and yoga instructor located in New York City, I advise, "Remember that choosing healthy choices is a means of practicing self-care. Food is not a reward, and exercise is not a punishment. Both of these are methods of taking care of your body and promoting your overall well-being. You merit them both.

Breathe In Deeply.
According to Hutchins, taking a few minutes to calm down and just concentrate on your breathing at the start of your exercise or even your day may help you set goals, connect with your body, and even lessen your body's stress reaction. One hand should be on your stomach, and the other should be on your chest while you lay on your back with your legs outstretched. According to Hutchins, you should take four deep breaths via your nose, hold them for two, and then take six more breaths through your mouth. The only hand that should rise or fall with each breath should be the one that is resting on your tummy.

Throw The Calendar Away.
When you're reducing weight in a healthy and long-lasting way, "Patience is also vital." Additionally, there is no need to become bogged down in a calendar of objectives in the future if you concentrate on achieving genuinely achievable goals, such as walking 10,000 steps every single day. Focus on the fresh objectives and possible accomplishments that each 24-hour period brings. Lovell continues by saying that you should be

prepared for roadblocks along the path. Everybody loses weight in a unique way. It's crucial to know how to handle disappointments and expectations in a constructive manner. This gives dieters an opportunity to stay committed to adopting good lifestyle choices, he says.

Decide What Your "Problem Ideas" Are.
Work to stop and alter the ideas that are causing you problems, when you gaze in the mirror, perhaps your inner conversation is the cause. or the want to eat when you're anxious. Whatever your specific troubling thoughts are, force them to end by saying "stop" aloud.

Although it may seem ridiculous, that straightforward action will interrupt your train of thinking and give you the chance to substitute a more positive notion for it. The easiest technique to do this is to count backwards from one to 100 as many times as necessary until the negative thoughts stop, a key component of implementing long-lasting habit modification is having a general awareness of your thoughts and how they affect your behavior. The more conscious we are of our ideas, the more able we are to determine whether they are constructive or destructive. Thoughts that aren't beneficial can block you from moving forward and prevent you from making long-lasting adjustments.

As you learn to recognize when you are thinking negatively, you may decide which ideas to focus on. Consider these concepts as radio dials: The goal is to turn down the volume of negative thoughts and turn up the volume of ones that help you achieve your goals. Always keep in mind that this procedure takes time and requires experience."

Reject the all-or-nothing mentality, many dieters "destroy their attempts to lose weight by adopting an all-or-nothing mindset." Many people try unrealistically rigorous food and exercise objectives, which causes them to veer off course within weeks or even days. Once off course, the cognitive process shifts to "I can't do this" or "This is too difficult. Vani advises putting greater emphasis "on complete wellness" to avoid slipping into that trap. Both mental and physical wellness are meant by this.

Keep Your Feet Off The Scale.
The scale isn't necessarily terrible, but many of us have come to link it with negative ideas and behaviors. If that describes you, delaying getting on the scale until you reach a point where it no longer determines your value.

A healthy weight consists of more than just a scale reading, finding alternative metrics for tracking your development aside from the scale. You could feel better after a healthy weight decrease. Awesome potential benefits of a healthy weight loss journey include the capacity to improve your attitude, make greater functional mobility feasible, boost your vitality, or alleviate pain or suffering.

A great approach to track your progress without ever stepping on the scale is by making little changes in these areas. Many individuals hold the false assumption that altering their weight on the scale would resolve all of their problems. But this is in a "losing scenario. "Put a stop to this," You should pay more attention to the process and the trip rather than just the outcome (the number on the scale). Instead of putting pressure on results, be sure to appreciate your efforts along the way because they are the result of your commitment to finishing the phases leading up to your end goal.

Talk To Yourself Like You Would A Friend.
"When it comes to how we see ourselves and how we see our bodies, we are fairly critical of ourselves. We have high expectations for ourselves. We wouldn't make many of those expectations of our friends or loved ones, either.

Additionally, note that "transformation is hard." The time and focus needed to effect real change are frequently in limited supply due to busy daily schedules. When things don't go as planned, be gentle to yourself and remember that you can still accomplish your goals despite the difficulties you face. Treat yourself with the dignity and kindness that you deserve from everyone.

Get Rid Of The Idea That Some Meals Are Good Or Bad.

We've developed the habit of feeling either proud of or guilty about every dietary decision we make. However, food is just that, and you shouldn't feel bad if you sometimes crave a cookie. "Allow yourself to have a glass of wine or some chocolate cake." Remember that every meal is appropriate. Food is food; having a cupcake every now and then does not make you a bad person or a failure.

Think On What Is Doable.

"If you've never worked out at a gym before, your objective shouldn't be to complete 30 minutes of elliptical training on the first day. A 20-minute stroll could be a better objective.

If you want to cook more but lack expertise with healthy recipes or don't have a lot of time, don't expect yourself to make brand-new healthy meals every evening after work. Consider utilizing a meal delivery service like HelloFresh or Blue Apron, which delivers proportioned ingredients and meals to your door and lets you experiment with new foods and recipes while honing your culinary skills.

Start Where You Are, Then Steadily Advance.
The body of the typical guy has 43.2 pounds of fat. And that number is never static; it is always either rising or falling at any given time. Over time, you'll permanently bury your stomach if you spend more time each day burning fat than accumulating it. Sound easy? It is. As you can see, there is no one magic trick to losing weight. In fact, if you locate 100 happy losers, they'll tell you 100 different techniques to speed up weight reduction and triumph over the bulge.

However, the 50 suggestions listed below are meant to help you lose weight more quickly (lose your love handles, bust your gut, and define your abs). You may burn off your fat more quickly and easily than you ever thought possible if you only add three or four of them into your daily routine.

CHAPTER TWO
50 STRATEGIES TO QUICKLY LOSE WEIGHT.

1.   Consume Extra Protein.
While just 6 to 8 percent of the calories in carbohydrates are expended during digestion, about 25 to 30 percent of the calories in each gram of protein are. Run the numbers: Every time you swap 50g of protein for 50g of carbohydrates, you save 41 calories.

2. Examine Labels
Avoid eating anything that has "high-fructose corn syrup" as an ingredient. Since 1971, the U.S. has seen a more than 350% growth in the usage of this sugar replacement, which is used to sweeten soda, commercial baked products, and even sauces.

3. Get Out Of My Way.
Every exercise should be performed standing up.

4. Vary Your Motions

When you lift, alternating sets of lower-body exercises with sets of upper-body exercises in supersets. In this manner, your upper body may operate while your lower body is at rest. According to Craig Ballantyne, C.S.C.S., "this enables you to engage your muscles fully with very little pause between sets for a quicker, more effective exercise."

5. Perform A Blind Exercise

Try releasing the handlebars and shutting your eyes while using the elliptical trainer. (Take care!) Your core muscles will have to work harder to keep you balanced without the visual cues, burning more calories and accelerating weight reduction.

6. Accept Yardwork

Look at each physical activity as an opportunity to train your body and burn fat, even ones you attempt to avoid, like mowing the grass. (Only be certain to use a push mower.)

7. Indulge In Some Dill Pickles.

Per slice, they contain one calorie. Man flipping a huge tire as a form of physical exercise

8. Move More Forcefully.

One out of every five steps should be skipped when utilizing the stair climber. After then, take a big step to resume your regular gait.C.S.C.S., this step increases muscle recruitment, hastening weight reduction.

9. Rent Incentives

Watch a movie that motivates you to work out once every week. Rocky (for the gym), American Flyers (for cycling), Hoosiers (for team sports), Chariots of

Fire, and Without Limits are a few examples (both for running).

10. Set A New Record

Every time you work out, set a goal to run a fraction of a mile longer in the same amount of time. This guarantees that from one workout to the next, you're burning more calories, which is essential for weight reduction.

11. Break Your Dinner Dishes, Then Get Smaller Ones.

In this manner, even if you completely load your plate, you still end up consuming less food than you would normally pour upon your current plates.

12. Reduce Carbohydrates

You have undoubtedly heard it countless times. Because it is effective. A Journal of Nutrition analysis indicated that men who cut their carb consumption to only 8% of their daily calories shed 7 pounds of fat and built 2 pounds of muscle in just six weeks. This is just one of several recent studies that support this claim.

13. Run After Lifting.

performing cardio after lifting weights—when you're already exhausted—will have a stronger impact than doing it beforehand.

14. Reverse Course

On the elliptical machine, try this interval training tip: Ride as quickly as you can for the first 30 seconds, then instantly change directions and ride for another 30 seconds as quickly in the opposite way. Repeat after a 60-second break. According to Alwyn Cosgrove, C.S.C.S., the power of stopping your momentum as well as going from a complete stop to full speed again in the same time would significantly increase your attempts to burn fat

15. Fill Up On Meals Strong In Fiber

Think of them as "healthy carbohydrates". Their size fills up your stomach, making you feel full and causing you to eat less. The best source of fiber is beans, which provide 8g in a half cup. According to research, men who increased their daily intake of fiber by 12 grams (g) had a quarter-inch loss in their love handles without changing anything else about their diet

16. Drizzle Vinaigrette Dressing On Top Of Your Salad.

In your body's fat incinerator, acidic meals like vinegar and lemon juice act as lighter fluid, accelerating carb burning by 20 to 40 percent, according to studies. According to researchers, the acids reduce insulin surges and slow down how quickly food leaves the stomach.

Pickles and yogurt, which have been fermented, are other excellent sour alternatives.

17. Avoid Skipping Meals

Long durations of fasting cause your body to enter a catabolic state, which causes it to start using fat instead of muscle for energy. While intermittent fasting may help you lose weight, skipping meals puts you in danger.

18. Make Use Of The Versaclimber

When practicing exercise, burning more calories depends on how vertical you are.

19. Avoid Staying In Bed All Day.

If you're a TV addict, tally up how many hours you watch each week, and stop watching any repeats—even if Seinfeld is on and you've never seen it. Spend the extra time on your feet by going outside or to the gym.

20. Work The Muscles.

If you're lazy, it's not as horrible as you think; three days a week of lifting for just 10 minutes will be beneficial. Harvard research demonstrates that weight exercise for 30 minutes per week has a higher impact on waist size reduction than practically any other factor.

21. Pass On The Potatoes, Please.

any form, including mashed, baked, French fries, and potato chips. They cause an increase in blood insulin levels, which causes your body to stop burning fat and start storing it instead. (Sweet potatoes are permitted since they are higher in fiber and minerals.)

22. *After Working Out, Eat Your Largest Meal Of The Day.*

To digest food, you need calories. And according to University of Nevada studies, processing meals after a weight-training session requires 73 percent more calories than it would have otherwise.

23. *Drink Water Before A Meal.*

According to Christopher Mohr, M.S., R.D., the water will take up space in your stomach, causing you to feel fuller and stifling your appetite.

24. *Request Replacements*

Ask for veggies whenever your restaurant dish includes a side of pasta, potatoes, or rice, (Your server will be delighted to make room for you.)

25. *Join A League.*

In other words, enroll in a sport like kickball, softball, or even soccer. Exercise sessions will be automatically scheduled into your week, and because you're on a team, peer pressure will make sure you keep going.

26. Break In Between Scoops.

That is, feel free to indulge in one scoop (about 1/2 cup) or one tiny piece of ice cream, cake, or any high-calorie dessert if you can't live without it. Wait 20 minutes, and if you still want more, do so. Usually, while you wait, hormones take effect and cause a sensation of fullness, which decreases the urge for that second dish.

27. Floss Your Teeth More Frequently.

Researchers from Japan have discovered that males who regularly washed their teeth were thinner than guys who did not in a study involving 14,000 participants. Thank goodness for the flavor, which may discourage you from snacking in between meals.

28. Eat An Imbalanced Diet.

You may maintain your metabolism active by rotating your caloric intake so that you consume more calories one day and less the next, and doing so will ensure that you continue to burn fat quickly. The secret is to aim for an average of 2,000 calories each day over the course of a week.

29. Turn The Incline Up.

When you run outside, you exert power on the ground and move ahead just with your bodyweight. The belt aids your running while you are on a treadmill. Always walk or run with at least a 1 percent inclination to avoid this problem; according to an English research, this treadmill grade is practically identical to running outside.

30. Limit Calorie-Free Beverages.
That includes water, coffee, tea, diet soda, and mixes like Crystal Light.

31. Consume Breakfast Each Day.
People who routinely eat breakfast had obesity rates that are 35 to 50% lower than those who don't, according to research from Harvard and Boston's Children's Hospital. Morning meals, according to nutritionists, help control appetite and insulin levels, reducing the likelihood that you'll overeat the rest of the day.

32. Steer clear of goods packaged in a bag or box.
These are often highly processed carbohydrates, which spike blood sugar levels fast and prevent your body from burning fat.

33. Between-Meal Snacks.
This not only prevents you from overeating at lunch and supper since you won't be ravenous, but it also makes your body metabolize food all day long, which boosts your metabolism and promotes weight reduction.

34. Records reflect.
And just view the programs you have recorded. You can minimize your TV watching—and the amount of time you spend on the couch—by more than a third by skipping the ads and just watching the shows you care about enough to get a season pass for.

35.Don't be afraid to try plain Greek yogurt.
When volunteers were randomly assigned to one of two diets, one high in calcium and the other not, and each group's caloric intake was reduced by 500 calories, researchers at the University of Tennessee discovered that those receiving calcium lost twice as much weight (an average of 13 pounds) as those on the standard diet. Extra calcium aids in increased fat metabolism and decreased fat storage.

36. Omit The Amuse-Bouche.
And stay far away from the bread bowl. If you are starving when you go to a restaurant, order a side salad or an appetizer that is simply made of meat or vegetables instead of giving in to the temptation of these bottomless—and fattening—freebies.

37.Popped Peanuts
Because they make you feel fuller after eating than many other meals, nuts have a very high satiety power. And even though they contain a lot of calories, the body seems to metabolize those calories in a different way. Researchers from the University of Michigan discovered that males who increased

their daily intake of peanuts by 500 calories did not experience any weight gain.

38. *Avoid Going Hungry*

a weight-loss researcher at the University of Michigan, "Under normal circumstances, humans absorb only approximately 80% of the nutrients from the food they eat." However, when the body is starved of food, it transforms into a super-efficient machine. gadget that extracts as many nutrients as it can from the food that is ingested. Your body might not catch up if you resume eating regularly; instead, it will keep storing food as fat.

39. *Perform Sprint Intervals*

The best cardio for losing weight consists of short, all-out sprints separated by brief rest intervals. Try a 2 to 1 "work-to-rest" ratio. In other words, run for two times as long as you rest. Therefore, after sprinting for 150 yards—a suitable starting distance—in 20 seconds, take a 10-second break, then repeat 3–7 times.

40. *Assess Your Emotional State*

It's possible that the want to snack is brought on by feelings of loneliness, despair, or worry rather than actual hunger. a psychotherapist in New York City, claims that emotional eating is at the root of poor eating decisions. An issue can exist if you frequently eat to make yourself feel better or if eating makes you happy.

41. Make A Purchase

Buy the single-serving packet rather than the big, family-style bag if you must purchase cookies, chips, or other processed junk food. In this manner, you will finally have far less harm done to your waistline when you consume the entire packet, which, let's be honest, you know you will.

42. Eat Slowly

it can take up to 12 minutes for the signal that you've started eating to get to your brain. Quick tip: Drink water in between bites of food or, at the very least, eat more meals with friends or family. You'll probably chat more as a consequence and eat slower as a result.

43. Go The Extra Mile

Instead of intervals at a certain period, do intervals for a specified distance. Otherwise, when you weary, you'll be doing shorter sprints, which will lower the quantity of calories you burn,

44. I Swindle Once A Week.

Use the dinner as a reward after a week of diligent labor or the conclusion of a challenging assignment, it's OK for you to skip one meal a week without feeling terrible." "If you eat healthily 95% of the time, you can relax and have fun the other 5% of the time without putting on weight."

45. Row Upwards

Every time you finish 10 repetitions on the rowing machine, raise the handles straight over your head for two repetitions in a row without bending your elbows. Then, switch back to your regular rowing form, this puts additional strain on your shoulders, back, and legs since they must exert more force to provide you the momentum to complete the exercise.

46. Avoid White Bread

Researchers from Tufts University examined the diets and waistlines of 459 individuals and discovered that even among males of same age and activity level, those who regularly ate white bread weighed more than those who didn't. According to this research calorie from white bread and refined grains just tend to settle at the waistline more than calories from other meals.

47. Pay Attention To Portion Quantities.

a professor in the University of Rhode Island's department of kinesiology, states that "the majority of people who have been thin their whole lives have a lot better awareness of optimal portion size than persons who are overweight." If they dine out, they are significantly more likely to leave food on their plate rather than cleaning it up or to request a doggy bag immediately away.

48. *You should never deny yourself a favorite cuisine.*

Here's a surprise: 30 ladies were instructed by a team of British researchers to stay away from chocolate before being placed in a room full of the substance compared to others who hadn't been given the command, women were far more likely to steal a taste. Blame the appeal of the forbidden: The more you tell yourself you're not allowed to consume something you enjoy, the more you'll desire it.

49. *Improve Yourself*

Try this interval routine when using a rowing machine: Row for 60 seconds, then rest for 60 seconds while noting the distance on the machine. Repeat, but this time row for 55 seconds and aim to equal or surpass your previous attempt's distance. Reduce the time to 50 seconds by repeating after a 55-second break. Continue until you are unable to surpass your starting distance.

50. *Use A Scale To Weigh Oneself Each Day.*

This is one habit that keeps coming up repeatedly with the thousands of patients enrolled in the registry, according to the originator of the National Weight Control Registry, which keeps track of almost 4,500 men and women who have shed at least 20 pounds and kept it off for at least six years on average. The recommendation is to "don't obsess over the number, but at least keep note of the range of what you weigh." You'll be able to notice little changes as they happen and react quickly to remedy them if you do this.

CHAPTER THREE

How can I permanently lose weight?

Your risk of coronary heart disease may be affected by your weight (CHD). Obesity, defined as a BMI of 30 or more, is a risk factor for CHD, but weight is also associated with other diseases including type 2 diabetes and high blood pressure.

Calculating your BMI might be a useful place to start if you're unsure of whether you need to lose weight or if your weight is healthy for your height. As your body form is crucial, measure your waist as well. Even if your BMI is within the safe range, carrying too much weight around your midsection raises danger.

Everyone wants to lose weight quickly when it comes to keeping it off, and there are a lot of diets out there that promise speedy results. Although they could be effective in the short term, they are frequently difficult to maintain, which causes the weight to soon regain.

To identify the sorts of crash diets that are best avoided, keep an eye out for some of these typical diet misconceptions and fads while selecting a diet.

The Following Are A Senior Dietitian's Top Recommendations For Weight Loss In A Healthy Way:

While changing eating patterns is a necessary part of losing weight, this shouldn't imply skipping meals or avoiding entire food categories. Aim for consistent mealtimes and a balanced diet, but be mindful of your portion amounts. You can be consuming a healthy variety of meals, but in excess. There are other factors to take into account besides just your diet. The best weight reduction strategies combine dietary adjustments with increased physical activity and address some of your eating-related behaviors to help you better understand your own eating habits and how you react to food under various conditions.

Diets that drastically restrict or exclude certain nutrient-dense foods or food groupings are not likely to be a long-term answer. While fad diets centered on specific items (cabbage soup, anyone?) encourage consuming a lot of one type of food and little of another, the more severe high-protein, low-carbohydrate diets restrict fruit, vegetables, and fiber, especially in the early phases. Some diets may severely restrict calorie consumption to help you see results quickly. An extremely low calorie intake, however, may cause you to get exhausted and hungry, which may lead you to give up and gain the weight back rapidly.

According to national recommendations, a daily calorie intake decrease of roughly 600 is required for long-term weight loss. This can result in a weekly weight loss of around 0.5 kg (1lb). Although it may not seem like much in comparison to the claims made by many quick-fix diets, it enables you to permanently adopt healthy eating habits into your lifestyle, increasing your likelihood of maintaining your weight loss. Woman choosing something to eat while perusing the refrigerator.

10 MORNING EXERCISES FOR LOSING WEIGHT.

Whatever your goals are for losing weight, it might occasionally seem difficult. But shedding a few pounds doesn't necessarily require making drastic dietary and lifestyle changes. In actuality, a few modest changes to your morning routine will help you lose weight and keep it off.

This chapter provides a list of 10 easy morning rituals you may adopt to help with weight reduction.

1. Consume A High-Protein Breakfast.
Breakfast is regarded as the most significant meal of the day for a reason, your morning meal can determine how the rest of the day will go. If you

need a mid-morning snack before heading to the vending machine or whether you'll be satisfied and full until lunch depends on this. A breakfast that is heavy in protein may reduce cravings and promote weight reduction.

In a research involving 20 teenage females, having a high-protein breakfast significantly decreased post-meal cravings compared to a low-protein breakfast.

Another small study found that, as compared to having a meal with standard protein, eating a high-protein breakfast was related with less fat accumulation, decreased day consumption, and decreased appetite. Protein may also aid in weight loss by reducing levels of ghrelin, the "hunger hormone" that increases appetite.

In fact, a high-protein meal reduced ghrelin release more efficiently than a high-carb breakfast did in a research involving 15 males. To help you start your day off correctly, think about eating protein-rich foods like eggs, Greek yogurt, cottage cheese, almonds, and chia seeds. A high-protein breakfast may help with weight reduction by lowering desires, hunger, and ghrelin release, according to studies.

2. Consume Lots Of Water
A simple strategy to improve weight reduction is to start your morning with one or two glasses of water. You can increase your energy expenditure or burn

more calories if you drink water for at least 60 minutes.

In a single, short research, consuming 16.9 fluid ounces (500 ml) of water resulted in an average rise in metabolic rate of 30%. According to a different research, overweight women who raised their daily water intake to over 34 ounces (one liter) over the course of a year lost an additional 4.4 pounds (2 kg) without changing their diet or exercise regimen.

Additionally, some people may experience a decrease in appetite and food consumption after drinking water. Drinking 16.9 fluid ounces (500 ml) of water at breakfast time lowered calorie intake by 13% in a study of 24 elderly people. In reality, the majority of research on the subject have revealed that consuming 34–68 ounces (1-2 liters) of water daily can help people lose weight.

Drinking water first thing in the morning and remaining hydrated all day long are wonderful ways to accelerate weight reduction with no effort. SYNOPSIS Increasing your water consumption has been linked to greater energy expenditure, weight loss, and a reduction in hunger and food intake.

3. Check Your Weight
Self-control and motivation may both be improved by stepping on the scale each morning and weighing

oneself. Numerous research has linked higher weight reduction and daily self-weighing.

For instance, a study of 47 participants indicated that those who measured themselves daily over the course of six months lost around 13 pounds (6 kg) more weight than those who did it less frequently. According to another research, during a two-year period, persons who weighed themselves daily shed an average of 9.7 pounds (4.4 kg), whereas those who did so once a month gained 4.6 pounds (2.1 kg).

Another way to encourage healthy habits and behaviors that can aid in weight loss is by weighing oneself each morning. Frequent self-weighing was linked to better restraint in one significant research. Additionally, individuals who ceased regularly weighing themselves were more likely to report an increase in calorie consumption and a decline in self-control.

When you first wake up, weigh yourself for the best results. Do this after using the restroom and before consuming any food or liquids.

Additionally, keep in mind that a number of things, including your everyday activities, might affect how much you weigh. Instead of getting caught up in minute daily changes, keep an eye out for general weight reduction patterns and concentrate on the broader picture. According to studies, self-weighing every day may lead to greater restriction and more weight reduction.

4. Enjoy The Sun

You may jumpstart your weight reduction by opening the curtains to allow in some light or by going outside for a few additional minutes each morning. One tiny research discovered that even low levels of light exposure at specific times of the day might affect weight.

In addition, a research on animals revealed that mice given a high-fat diet were less likely to acquire weight when exposed to UV light.

Sunlight exposure is the best approach to provide your body with the vitamin D it needs. Getting adequate vitamin D may aid in weight loss or possibly prevent weight gain, according to several research.

218 overweight and obese women participated in one trial, taking vitamin D supplements or a placebo for a full year. At the end of the trial, individuals who consumed the recommended amount of vitamin D lost an average of 7 pounds (3.2 kg) more weight than those whose blood levels of the vitamin were insufficient. A different investigation that tracked 4,659 older women for four years discovered a correlation between greater vitamin D

levels and decreased weight gain Your skin type, the time of year, and your location may all affect how much sun you need. However, allowing in some sunlight or spending a few minutes each morning outside may help with weight reduction. The weight you carry might be affected by sun exposure. Getting enough vitamin D from the sun may aid in accelerating weight reduction and preventing weight gain.

5. Engage In Mindfullness
The practice of mindfulness is being completely present in the moment and being mindful of your thoughts and feelings, It has been demonstrated that the technique enhances weight reduction and encourages wholesome eating practices.

For instance, a review of 19 trials revealed that mindfulness-based therapies improved weight reduction and decreased eating habits associated with obesity. Similar results were found in another analysis, which noted that 68 percent of the research looked at showed a substantial weight loss as a result of mindfulness training, being aware is easy to do. Start by allocating five minutes each morning to rclax in a serene area and open your senses. According to some study, mindfulness can promote responsible eating habits and help people lose weight.

6. Fit In A Little Exercise

The weight reduction benefits of exercising first thing in the morning can be increased. In one study, the benefits of aerobic exercise at various times of the day were evaluated in 50 overweight women.

Exercise in the morning was linked to a higher degree of satiety, despite there being little change in particular food desires between individuals who exercised in the morning vs the afternoon. Exercise in the morning could also help keep your blood sugar levels steady all day. One of the various negative symptoms of low blood sugar is an excessive hunger. Working exercise in the morning was linked to better blood sugar management, according to one research including 35 individuals with type 1 diabetes. These investigations, however, were relatively narrowly targeted and only found a correlation, not a causal relationship. The benefits of early exercise on the general population require further study.

Exercise in the morning has been linked to enhanced satiety and better blood sugar regulation, according to certain research.

7. Bring A Lunch.

Planning and packing your lunch in advance can be a quick and easy approach to improve dietary choices and accelerate weight reduction. Meal planning was linked to a better quality diet, greater diversity in food, and a decreased risk of obesity, according to a major study including 40,554 participants

According to a different study, eating more home-cooked meals on a regular basis was linked to better diet quality and a lower chance of having too much body fat. In fact, compared to people who only ate home-cooked meals three times or fewer per week, those who ate them at least five times per week were 28% less likely to be overweight. To make it easier to take your lunch and leave in the morning, try blocking out a few hours one evening per week to plan and prepare your meals.

Research indicates that meal planning and consuming home-cooked food are linked to better diet quality and a decreased risk of obesity.

8. Get More Rest
Try going to bed earlier or delaying your alarm if you want to sleep for a few extra hours. Numerous studies have discovered that a lack of sleep may be linked to an increase in hunger. One small study indicated that sleep deprivation enhanced desires for high-calorie, high-carb meals and increased hunger.

Lack of sleep has also been linked to an increase in calorie intake. In one study, 12 volunteers found that after only four hours of sleep, they devoured, on average, 559 more calories than they did after eight hours. Along with eating healthily and exercising, getting into a regular sleep routine is essential for weight reduction. Aim for at least eight hours of sleep each night to get the best outcomes. SYNOPSIS Research suggests that lack of sleep may lead to an increase in calorie consumption, hunger, and desires.

9. Alternate Your Commute.

Driving may not be the healthiest method to go to work, while being one of the most convenient options. According to research, taking public transit, bicycling, or walking may lower body weight and lessen the risk of weight gain. According to a research that tracked 822 people for four years, those who commuted by automobile tended to gain more weight than those who didn't.

Similar to this, a research including 15,777 participants found that utilizing active transportation, such as walking or bicycling, was linked to a lower body mass index and body fat percentage than using private transportation. The mere act of switching up your commute, even a few times a week, might help you lose weight more quickly. Compared to driving to work, taking public transit, walking, riding, and biking have all been linked to decreased body weight and body fat.

10. Begin Monitoring Your Intake.
A good strategy to promote weight reduction and hold yourself responsible is to keep a food diary to record what you consume. One study followed 123 participants' weight loss over the course of a year and discovered that keeping a food record was linked to better weight reduction.

Another study revealed that individuals lost more weight when they utilized a monitoring device to routinely monitor their diet and activity than when they did not.

Similarly, a study of 220 obese women found that using a self-monitoring tool often and consistently enhanced long-term weight control. Consider utilizing an app or even just a pen and paper to keep a food and beverage log starting with your first meal of the day. SYNOPSIS Research has shown that keeping a food journal to monitor your consumption helps speed up weight reduction. Your morning routine may be easily and effectively changed in order to accelerate weight reduction.

CHAPTER FOUR
STRATEGIES TO NAVIGATE THROUGH THE WEIGHT LOSS PATH.

Creating healthy morning routines can assist you in getting off to a good and positive start each day. For best results, be sure to combine these morning rituals with a healthy diet and an active way of life. You might be concerned that you'll have to give up eating all of your favorite meals if you're attempting to lose a few pounds. However, eliminating some items from your diet entirely might actually boost cravings and make it more difficult to control your weight. You may still enjoy eating in moderation by adjusting when and how you eat. We'll start with meal adjustments, then move on to additional strategies you might use to curb your appetite and support your weight reduction goals.

Observe Portion Sizes.

Smaller portions help you better manage your calorie intake.

Your diet accounts for the bulk of weight reduction. Pay attention to the serving suggestions and nutritional facts on the container rather than stuffing your face with everything on your plate. You don't have to exclude some foods entirely from your diet, but you should try to limit your intake to one serving at a time and wait to see how you feel afterward before consuming more. Suitable serving sizes include

roughly the size of a deck of cards, a dish of beef.

a tennis ball-sized portion of fruit

the equivalent of a baseball-sized serving of veggies

a dish of carbohydrates the size of a hockey puck, such as pasta or rice

a pair of dice-sized serving of fats

Consume protein and fiber together with your favorite foods.

Both protein and fiber make you feel fuller. Whole-grain breads and pastas, broccoli, carrots, apples, and bananas are a few foods that are rich providers of fiber. For an additional 7–11 grams of fiber per serving, add chia or basal seeds to sauces or smoothies. The healthiest sources of protein include lean meats, nuts, beans, and legumes.

Try to consume between 46 and 56 grams of protein and between 21 and 38 grams of fiber per day.

To assist you curb your hunger even more, add some red pepper or spice to your meals.

Try to include foods with no added sugars and more than 3 grams of fiber per serving.

Eat slowly to avoid overeating.

Eat more slowly so you can recognize when you are full. Take smaller bits when you eat and put your fork down while you chew so you won't feel the need to take more. In between mouthful, assess your level of satisfaction and quit eating if necessary. a lack of hunger. Save any remaining food on your plate rather than making yourself consume it right now. [7] Typically, it takes 20 minutes until you feel satisfied. Try taking a little rest before eating more if you want seconds. [8] To increase your feeling of fullness, take the time to appreciate the flavor of your food with each bite.

You'll forget to pay attention to whether you're full if you watch TV or engage in other distractions while eating.

Do not eat when you are bored.

Eat only when you are actually hungry. Since eating makes you feel more comfortable, you tend to eat more when you're feeling sad or bored. Consider whether you genuinely need food and are hungry. Instead of eating when you don't feel like it, consider taking a stroll, phoning a friend, or visiting the gym to keep yourself occupied. To assist you overcome any desires for food while you're bored, try chewing a piece of sugar-free gum.

Note the cuisine you're desiring as well as your current mood. You're more likely to pinpoint the factors that lead to your overeating once you've written it down on paper.

Hide the less healthy selections.

You'll consume fewer problem foods if you hide them in awkward places. Put your chips and cookies on a higher shelf or store them in a different cupboard if you often graze on them throughout the day. Keep healthy alternatives around so you'll be more inclined to go for them when you need a fast snack, such as apples, bananas, or carrots.

Healthy substitutes should be stored in clear plastic wrap, while unhealthy items should be transferred into opaque containers or aluminum foil wraps. You are more inclined to choose the healthier alternative as you can see it clearly.

Place the food in a dish or on a plate.

If you eat straight from the package, you run the risk of overeating. When you munch straight from the container, it's more difficult to keep track of portion sizes and how much you've consumed. Instead, measure out the appropriate serving amount from the box and pour it into a bowl or plate. After eating a portion, you may always add more to your plate if you're still a little puckish.

Use more compact plates.

Filling your plate to the brim requires less food and aids with portion control. Instead of selecting your largest plate and filling it to the brim, choose for one that is somewhat smaller or has a broader rim. You won't have as large of portion sizes and are therefore less prone to overeat because your meal occupies more space on the smaller plate. Since studies have shown that placing unhealthy meals on a red plate may cause you to consume less food, try doing so to quell your appetites, savor your nibbles. Treating yourself once in a while is OK, but take your time. Purchase your preferred delicacy, indulge in little nibbles, savor the flavors, and store some for later. You'll consume them with greater satisfaction and experience fewer cravings as a result.

Arrange your meals in advance.

Choose a few meals to prepare so you can anticipate them. Search for a few recipes that you want to make this week. To avoid having to figure it out later, write down the days you'll eat each meal in a notepad or meal planner. After that, prepare a list of everything you need to buy and stick to it by just purchasing what you'll need for the coming week. You may always prepare all of your meals in bulk in advance and freeze the extra pieces for later reheating.

When you are hungry, you are more likely to buy items that aren't on your list at the grocery store.

Up your water intake.

Drinking water before and during meals might make you feel more satisfied. Avoid sugary drinks since they are high in calories and might prevent you from losing weight. Get a full glass of water before you sit down to eat. Drink few sips in between bites of food to make you feel fuller faster.

In moderation, soda and other sweet drinks are acceptable, but try switching to plain water for the majority of your daily hydration needs.

every day, spend 30 minutes exercising

By burning more calories than you ingest, you can lose weight. Make time during your day to engage in cardiovascular activities like walking, running, riding, or swimming. If you don't have time for a complete 30-minute workout, break it up into 10-minute segments throughout the day so you can get some of the calories you've consumed burned off.

Look for strategies to burn calories in your daily activities. Instead of taking the elevator, think about utilizing the stairs.

Exercise your muscles two times every week.

Fat burns less calories than muscle tissue. Set aside two days each week for bodyweight workouts, resistance band training, or weightlifting. These activities will assist increase your metabolism so it's easier to enjoy your regular diet, even though they will help you gain muscle more than they will help you lose fat.

Push-ups, sit-ups, squats, and dumbbell bicep curls are a few simple workouts you can perform at home.

Change the muscle groups you work out with each session to avoid becoming tired or straining your muscles. You may, for instance, train your arms and upper body one day while concentrating on your legs and core the next day.

Include some enjoyable new workouts

To reduce weight, you don't necessarily need to go to the gym. Look for local programs or activities that will keep you moving and active. Find out if there are any dance or Zumba classes available so you can work out to upbeat music. You may also try rollerblading, taekwondo, rock climbing, ice skating, or a pick-up game of your preferred sport. Simply look at the opportunities your neighborhood recreation or community center has to offer. Basketball games may help you burn 600–900 calories in only one hour!

Regularly stretch while standing up.

Your metabolism might slow down if you sit for a long time. Try to stand up for a few minutes every hour to stretch your legs if you spend most of your time sitting at a desk or leading a somewhat sedentary lifestyle. To feel revitalized, have a drink of water, go for a little office stroll, or practice some fast office yoga.

Long periods of sitting can inhibit the synthesis of lipase, an enzyme that aids in the breakdown of fats in the body.

Exercise relaxation techniques.

If you're anxious, you're more prone to overeat. Never eat comfort food when you're feeling a little tense or anxious.

Instead, identify what caused your feelings and search for strategies to prevent or control them. To calm your mind and get rid of any stress-inducing thoughts, try some deep breathing exercises, self-massage, or yoga. Try inhaling for four counts through your nose, holding your breath for seven counts, then gently expelling through your mouth for eight counts as a simple breathing exercise.

Have a restful night's sleep.

When you stay awake, your body requires more food for energy. You might not have the stamina to stay up if you typically feel hungry at night.

Try going to bed at a regular hour every night rather than caving to your desires. To feel less worried, more energized, and less hungry, try to obtain between 7-9 hours of sleep each night.

Frequent questions I get asked and My Answers.

Can junk food be consumed when losing weight?
A total calorie deficit is necessary to lose weight. Yes, you can lose weight by eating two bags of chips every day, but you won't receive the essential vitamins, minerals, protein, good fats, and carbohydrates, and you'll feel crappy.

Question

What foodstuffs are best for weight loss?
A calorie deficit is necessary for weight loss. Consume entire foods, including grains, legumes, fruits, and vegetables. Avoid eating or drinking anything that is packaged or in a box.

Question

Eat three meals a day, and can you still lose weight?
Yes, you can lose weight despite eating three meals a day as long as your daily calorie consumption is lower.

Question

If you eat a lot, is it possible to lose weight?
Yes, you can eat a lot if you avoid things high in calories like veggies.

Warnings

The FDA does not regulate dietary supplements; therefore, you should avoid taking them to burn calories.

Attempt to shed no more than 1-2 pounds (0.45-0.91 kg) each week. More rapid weight loss in a week might have negative health effects.

CHAPTER FIVE

You can eat everything you want and still lose weight.

You might believe that in order to reach and maintain a healthy weight, you must stop enjoying your favorite foods. That's not the case, though. You may indulge in your preferred cuisine while still losing weight.

Here is a brief guide on eating sensibly while giving in to your cravings.

Portion Management

Portion management is arguably the most crucial step in allowing yourself to consume the foods you enjoy. You'll learn all about wholesome portion proportions in the New Mayo Clinic Diet program. Finding out what a proper portion size is may be an eye-opening experience, albeit it may take some getting accustomed to. And if you start eating the appropriate foods—in the correct amounts—and start exercising portion control, you'll soon realize that a modest dish of your favorite indulgence is all you need. Throughout the course of the program, you'll learn strategies that can help you curb your appetite. For instance:

Avoid eating food directly from the packaging, since this makes it far too simple to nibble on many portions. Dish out a single meal instead, and then tuck the packet away.

Enjoy The Taste
When you consume your favorite foods, try to slow down and allow yourself to truly appreciate the moment, enjoying each and every bite, rather than chowing down on them in thoughtless gulps. Another skill you'll acquire in the New Mayo Clinic Diet program is mindful eating with a piece of chocolate, you may enjoy a tasty approach to practice mindful eating:

Take one little meal at a time while sitting down. Before swallowing, let each bite sit in your mouth for a few seconds. Take note of the overwhelming sweetness, creamy texture, and rich taste, You might be amazed by how one tiny piece of chocolate, when enjoyed carefully, can fulfill a sugar desire.

Include Exercise And Movement In Your Day.
Numerous health advantages of exercise include stress reduction, cognitive enhancement, and improved sleep. The acceleration of your calorie burn, however, is the true benefit when it comes to weight control. You are able to sometimes indulge in a favorite dish when you are desiring it since you know you are burning a few extra calories. Choose a regular physical activity and stick to it. Exercise can aid with weight reduction, happiness, and developing the proper mentality for choosing

healthier foods. There are several excellent activities you may perform at home.

Initially, fill up on fruits and veggies.
Fruits and vegetables may be wonderful additions to the cuisine you enjoy. They don't just have few calories; they also make you feel full and content. Therefore, always strive to load up on healthy foods by starting with vegetables and fruits when it comes to maintaining a balance in your nutrition. Eat a nutritious dinner first and reserve the sweets for dessert rather than indulging in your favorite confectionery on an empty stomach. You could consume less sweets. Additionally, by keeping the sugar for after your meal, you'll lessen the chance of a blood sugar spike. You may live the healthiest version of your life by including more fruits and vegetables into your diet. A brand-new, interactive habit optimizer is a feature of The New Mayo Clinic Diet that makes creating better habits, like this one, enjoyable.

Prepare your favorite dishes healthily.
Sometimes, your favorite comfort meals just require a few little adjustments to transform into healthier—yet equally delicious—versions of oneself. For instance, you may think about altering the way you prepare some ingredients: Try air-frying food as an alternative to deep-frying it! By substituting healthy elements for what you're seeking, you may

also elevate it: Consider using fruit instead of sugar as a source of sweetness while baking. All you require is an open mind and the desire to try new things in the kitchen.

The bottom line: Balance is key if you want to keep eating the things you enjoy while still losing weight. Everything in moderation is sound counsel that works, despite its trite appearance. You may have your cake and eat it too if you do it slowly, carefully, and in small portions. This will help you form a better, more lasting relationship with food. When you can no longer resist the cake, choosing to follow deprivation diets and foregoing all your favorite meals will only result in weight gain.

With no foods off-limits, The New Mayo Clinic Diet teaches you how to balance your nutrition. You'll discover how to include your favorite meals and develop a lifelong strategy for wellbeing.

The Best Foods for Losing Weight Healthily

All sizes and types of healthy bodies are possible. Even while weight reduction is not a panacea for health and not everyone needs to seek it, you might want to work toward it if you want to feel the healthiest.

If you mix a healthy diet with regular exercise, your diet can affect your health outcomes. (But get medical advice first before making any substantial changes!)

According to research, these 18 foods may encourage a healthy weight reduction journey if losing weight is your objective. Scientists' investigations have shown that some meals could affect appetite. When included in a nutritious diet and lifestyle, they may help with weight loss. Continue reading to find out more about seven meals that might aid in weight loss.

If someone wants to reduce weight, they should buy foods that are high in nutrients. Foods high in fiber and protein may be especially beneficial for controlling weight. Several foods, including fruits, vegetables, nuts, whole grains, and yogurt, have been linked to weight loss.

Potato chips, sweetened drinks, red meats, and processed meats were all linked to weight increase in the same research. These results suggest that while trying to lose weight, it may be better to restrict fried foods, foods with added sugar, high-fat meats, and processed foods.

Physical exercise is crucial for weight loss and maintaining weight loss, even though eating the correct meals may be helpful. A doctor should be consulted before beginning any physical exercise program.

CHAPTER SIX

SELECTING MEALS TO REDUCE WEIGHT

People ought to choose for baked, broiled, or grilled items rather than fried ones. Beans, chicken, eggs, fish, and turkey are examples of lean proteins that are suitable replacements for high-fat meats.

Even while picking healthy foods for weight reduction, it's crucial to pay attention to portion sizes.

Although they might contain a lot of calories, sugar-sweetened drinks do not make you feel as satisfied as solid foods do. Juice and soda should be substituted with calorie-free liquids like water or unsweetened tea

Added Helpful Weight Loss Advice
A crucial component of weight loss is exercise. Adults should exercise for 30 minutes five days a week, or 150 minutes every week, according to the American College of Sports Medicine. Before beginning a new exercise regimen, people should see their doctor.

Instead than focusing just on the weight on the scales, concentrate on making healthy changes. Smaller goals could seem less daunting than a single huge one. Although they might contain a lot of calories, sugar-sweetened drinks do not make you feel as satisfied as solid foods do. Juice and soda should be substituted with calorie-free liquids like water or unsweetened tea.

Instead than focusing just on the weight on the scales, concentrate on making healthy changes. Smaller goals could seem less daunting than a single huge one Along with making healthy dietary choices and maintaining an active lifestyle, focus on getting enough sleep and controlling your stress levels because both have an impact on your health.

Salmon
Salmon and other fatty fish are wonderfully nourishing and filling.

Salmon is a rich source of high-quality protein, beneficial lipids, and several critical elements. That combination can keep you full and assist you in achieving a healthier weight.

Omega-3 fatty acids, which are abundant in salmon, may help lessen inflammation. Obesity and metabolic disorders are both significantly influenced by inflammation. Additionally, fish and seafood in general may contain a sizable quantity of iodine.

The vitamin is required for healthy thyroid function, which is vital to maintain a healthy metabolism.

However, research indicates that a sizable portion of people do not meet their iodine requirements. You can get adequate iodine by increasing the amount of fatty fish in your diet.

Other fatty fish, such as mackerel, trout, sardines, herring, tuna, and others, are also very good for your health.

Tuna
Another filling, high-protein dish is tuna.

It's a lean fish, so it contains good fats and protein to keep you satisfied. Docosahexaenoic acid (DHA), an omega-3 fatty acid, is one of these good fats that may be good for your heart. Eating fish, particularly fatty fish like salmon and tuna, may be a fantastic way to improve your protein intake and provide your eyes and brain with healthy fish fats.

If you want to consume less calories, pick tuna variants that are canned in water. Oil-packed tuna has more calories, fat, and salt but could also be more satisfying. Depending on your demands that particular day.

Eggs
Recently, whole eggs have gained in popularity despite their widespread dislike due to their high cholesterol level. These worries sprang from misconceptions that overlooked how your body regulates cholesterol levels. Your body obtains it

from your diet or your liver as needed to maintain its baseline levels.

Moderate egg consumption, or 7 to 12 eggs per week, has been demonstrated to be safe for most people, however those who already have high levels of LDL (bad) cholesterol should be very careful about how much cholesterol they consume. Eggs are one of the healthiest meals to eat if you're trying to attain or maintain a healthier weight, even if a larger diet of eggs may increase LDL cholesterol levels in certain people.

Eggs are very nutrient-dense foods. Interestingly, although while egg whites provide 4-6 grams of protein apiece, practically all of its nutrients, including choline and vitamin D, are concentrated in the yolks.

This is crucial because, if you pay attention to your body's internal fullness and hunger cues, you may be able to reach or maintain a healthy weight. To put it another way, making it a habit to only eat when you're hungry and stop when you're full will help you lose weight.

In contrast to cereal, milk, and orange juice, eating eggs and buttered toast for breakfast boosted feelings of satiety (fullness) over the following four hours, according to a research including 50 healthy persons with higher weight. An egg-based breakfast that was high or moderate in both protein and fiber was associated with greater feelings of fullness than low fiber cereal and milk, according to another research of 48 healthy people.

Eating eggs may assist your weight reduction objectives while also providing you with a wealth of nutritious ingredients, since feeling satisfied may help prevent overeating triggered by feeling too hungry.

Popular foods like eggs, especially for breakfast, may aid with weight reduction. Researchers evaluated the impact of eating eggs versus a bagel for breakfast on food intake, hunger, and pleasure in a short trial with 21 women.

They also examined the levels of ghrelin, also known as the hunger hormone, blood sugar, and insulin.

Women who had eaten the egg breakfast consumed considerably less food at their next meal and over the course of the next 24 hours than those who had had the bagel breakfast, the researchers discovered.

Three hours after breakfast, individuals who had eaten the eggs felt fuller and less hungry than those who had eaten the bagel. The egg group had lower ghrelin levels than the bagel group after breakfast, as well as less of a shift in their blood sugar and insulin levels.

Oatmeal
A cup of oats first thing in the morning could also help you weigh less.

In a research Trusted Source including 47 individuals, it was examined if eating oatmeal as compared to a ready-to-eat breakfast cereal affected participants' appetite, feelings of fullness, and how much food they consumed at their next meal.

Participants who ate oatmeal felt noticeably fuller and less hungry than those who ate the cereal. Additionally, they consumed less calories at lunch after eating oatmeal than after morning cereal. The oatmeal had more protein, more fiber, and less sugar than the cereal while having the same number of calories as it did.

The scientists came to the conclusion that the results were likely caused by the different types of fiber, particularly a soluble fiber known as beta-glucan.

Lentils, Peas, Chickpeas, And Other Legumes
The broad group of pulses includes peas, beans, lentils, and chickpeas. Due to their protein and fiber content, effects on satiety and feeling full, they may have an impact on weight loss. Like oatmeal, pulses contain soluble fiber, which may cause digestion and absorption to take longer. Satiety-indicating hormones are released after a protein meal.

Studies that examined how ingesting pulses affected weight reduction were examined by researchers.

Significantly more weight was eliminated compared to diets lacking pulses. In comparison to diets without pulses, weight loss occurred on weight maintenance diets that did.

Legumes like beans and other legumes can help you lose weight. They include kidney beans, black beans, lentils, and a variety of other beans.

These foods usually have high quantities of fiber and protein, two nutrients that promote satiety. Frequently, they also include some resistant starch

Because of their high fiber content, beans might make some individuals feel bloated and gassy. However, careful preparation might lessen these negative effects. Consider purchasing dried beans and soaking them for several hours prior to cooking.

Lean Meats And Chicken Breast
For many, the meat food category is still debatable.

Beyond concerns with ethics and sustainability, it is still unknown if or how red meat increases the risk of heart disease or diabetes.

There is little proof that eating meat affects health outcomes, according to research. It can be difficult to understand this phrase, and it's sometimes taken to suggest that eating more meat is a good idea, but it actually only means that there isn't enough data to determine if it has a negative impact on health.

However, consuming a lot of red and processed meat raises your chances of developing cancer, diabetes, heart disease, and dying too soon.

Consuming fruits, vegetables, and whole grains combined with unprocessed meat in moderation (i.e., 2-3 servings per week) may help reduce some of the cancer risks connected with meat intake.

Both chicken and red meat are high in protein and iron when it comes to nutrition. Lean red meat cuts with less saturated fat than other cuts include skinless, high-protein flank steak and tenderloin. Choose them the majority of the time to enhance weight management and heart health more successfully. According to some theories, inflammation, which is linked to chronic illness, is fueled by saturated fat. However, this research has also produced some contradictory results.

The results of your diet might also have an impact on your health.

When red meat is cooked at high temperatures for an extended period of time—by smoking or grilling, for example—fat drippings are produced. These create a carcinogenic byproduct known as polycyclic aromatic hydrocarbons (PAHs) when they come into contact with hot cooking surfaces your exposure to smoking, clean up spills, and consume lean meat in moderation to lower your risk. This implies a weekly limit of a few 3-ounce (85-gram) meals. A serving is around the size of your hand's palm.

Nuts

A weight reduction diet supplemented with 50 grams (g) of almonds per day was compared to a weight loss diet devoid of nuts in a research Trusted Source including overweight and obese women. Those in the almond group lost a lot more weight than women in the nut-free group after three months.

Additionally, women in the almond group significantly reduced their blood sugar, total cholesterol, triglycerides, body mass index (BMI), and waist circumference. Protein and fiber are included in nuts, which may assist to explain how they affect body weight. They also include additional advantageous nutrients and heart-healthy lipids. Although nuts may be a part of a nutritious diet, moderation is still necessary because they are an energizing item.

After losing weight, people frequently worry about gaining it back.

In a significant study conducted in Europe, researchers discovered that over a 5-year period, persons who ate the most nuts acquired less weight than those who did not. Additionally, they were less likely to become overweight or obese.

Nuts are a high-fat food that also contains fiber, protein, and other plant chemicals that are good for your heart. Given that they provide proportionate levels of protein, fiber, and healthy fats, they are great snacks. Nut consumption has been linked to better metabolic health and even weight loss, according to studies.

Additionally, research on the general population have revealed that individuals who consume nuts often obtain more nutrients and maintain a healthier weight than those who do not.

You should be careful to eat only until you feel full when consuming this cuisine, as you do with any high-fat food. So, if your objective is to reduce weight, be mindful of your portion proportions. At first, try eating a handful of unsalted nuts. Then, in 15 to 20 minutes, check how you're feeling. Give yourself some time to digest and try half of another handful if you're still hungry.

Avocados
Avocados are a fruit that offer a variety of vitamins, minerals, fiber, and healthy fats. Additionally, they could support weight control.

According to a study of American adults, individuals who ate avocado regularly lost a lot of weight and had a lower BMI than those who did not. People who consumed avocados also had a tendency to consume more fruits, vegetables, and fiber than those who did not. Overall, the diets of individuals who ate avocados were healthier, and they consumed a lot less added sugar than those who didn't. They also had a decreased chance of developing metabolic syndrome than people who did not eat avocado.

Berry
Berries frequently rank among the fruits with the greatest fiber content, which has been related to weight control.

Each cup of blackberries or raspberries has 8 g of fiber. Berries may be included in a variety of dishes, including oatmeal, yogurt, and salads.

Vegetables with crucifers
Broccoli, cauliflower, cabbage, and Brussels sprouts are examples of cruciferous vegetables that contain fiber that may aid in weight loss.

They are ideal for achieving or maintaining a healthy weight thanks to a number of characteristics. For instance, they include minerals and fiber that keep you hydrated and satisfied. Additionally, leafy greens include thylakoids, plant substances that have been connected to improved appetite control and enhanced fullness in at least two human studies.

The participants in both trials took a 5-gram thylakoid supplement, which is equivalent to around 3.5 ounces (100 grams) of raw spinach. It is important to note, however, that both studies are small. Those who took the supplement, even only one dosage, reported improved hunger control and weight reduction.

The effectiveness of thylakoids derived from food sources as a strategy for reaching a healthy weight — as well as their long-term impacts in supplement form — still need more study in people. Meanwhile, leafy greens are virtually always an excellent complement to your diet because they include a variety of fiber and minerals.

You might feel fuller for longer and have fewer cravings for less nourishing meals by increasing your intake of leafy greens. Your longer-term, healthy weight loss objectives can be helped by developing a response to your body's natural indications of hunger and fullness.

You should see a healthcare provider or a qualified dietitian about how many servings of leafy greens you should consume each day if you take drugs, such as blood thinners like warfarin (Coumadin).

Vitamin K, which is abundant in leafy greens and may interfere with your medicine, the key is regular vitamin K consumption.

6 g of fiber, or 24 percent of the daily need for fiber, may be found in one cup of cooked Brussels sprouts. Avocados are a special kind of fruit because, unlike most other fruits, they are heavy in healthful fats rather than carbohydrates. They have particularly high levels of the monounsaturated oleic acid found in olive oil. Despite having a high fat content, avocados are also quite satiating due to their high water and fiber content. Additionally, studies suggest that their fat content can improve the amount of carotenoid antioxidants your body gets from plants, making them the ideal complement to salads made primarily of veggies. Actually, it might boost absorption by 4.6–12.6 times.

In fact, they aid in the absorption of other crucial fat-soluble vitamins (vitamins A, D, E, and K). In addition, avocados are a great source of potassium and fiber.

It's important to remember that avocados are high in energy, so if weight reduction is your aim, portion control is essential. The more you practice listening to your body's natural cues for hunger and fullness, the more instinctively you can determine what the ideal serving size is for you at that particular moment.

Potatoes And Other Root Vegetables
The popularity of reduced carb diets may be at least partially to blame for the apparent decline in demand for white potatoes. For what it's worth, potatoes and other root vegetables offer a number of benefits that make them excellent sources of nutrients for promoting healthy weight reduction. They include a small amount of practically every nutrient you require and a very wide variety of nutrients.

Potassium, a nutrient that is generally underutilized, is particularly abundant in them. Potassium has a key role in blood pressure regulation. The Satiety Index, a system that determines how satisfied one feels after eating different foods, gave boiling white potatoes the highest grade of any item tested.

This implies that eating cooked white or sweet potatoes increases the likelihood that you will naturally feel satisfied afterward. Additionally, you'll be giving your body the nutrition it needs. After boiling, potatoes will produce large levels of resistant starch, a material that resembles fiber and has been linked to a number of health advantages, including weight loss.

Other wonderful options include sweet potatoes, turnips, and other root vegetables.

Soups

Eating more soup may be a delightful way to improve your diet of healthy grains and veggies, something you might not do otherwise. However, cream-based soups and variants that use processed meats won't offer the same nutritious benefit. Some people take longer to eat soup than other dishes because of the slurping, sniffing, tasting, chilling, and chewing. You could eat more deliberately if you eat more slowly. It could also aid in preventing overeating. Reaching and maintaining a healthy weight depend on you feeling full and nourishing your body while paying attention to and acting on your body's hunger and fullness cues.

There are methods to make soup creamier without using heavy cream, which can contribute less beneficial saturated fat, if you like a richer soup. Consider mixing in avocado, which enhances your soup's fiber content, or cashews. You may also garnish the soup with sliced avocado. Soups might help you feel fuller and control your weight because they are naturally watery and hydrate you. Including a vegetable-based clear soup before a meal will help you feel fuller and shed pounds in a healthy way.

Beware

When it comes to nutrition, trying to "do it properly" may seem alluring, but it might backfire.

Consider asking for help if you frequently follow restrictive diets, are always worried about your weight or food, feel guilty about your dietary decisions, or are concerned with these issues. These actions might be a sign of an eating disorder or a disturbed relationship with food.

No matter a person's gender identity, color, age, financial background, or other identities, disordered eating and eating disorders can impact them.

They are not just brought on by exposure to diet culture; they may also be brought on by any combination of biological, social, cultural, and environmental variables.

If you're having trouble, don't be afraid to speak with a licensed healthcare provider, such a registered dietitian.

The National Eating Disorders Association hotline also offers free online chat, free phone calls, and free texts with professional volunteers, as well as access to its free and low-cost resources.

Cottage Cheese
Protein content is often high in dairy products.

Cottage cheese, which is mainly protein, is one of the dairy products with the highest protein content.

You may increase your protein intake, which is crucial for developing and maintaining muscle, by eating cottage cheese. Additionally, it is abundant in calcium and quite filling. The association between calcium consumption and a healthy weight may perhaps exist, although more study is required in this area. Greek yogurt and skyr are two more dairy products with a high protein content.

wholesome grains

A diet high in whole grains, according to recent studies, can assist healthy weight loss. Cereal grains may be nutritious additions to your diet and may be good for your metabolism. That is as a result of their high fiber and respectable protein content. A few examples include quinoa, brown rice, and oats. Oats include a lot of soluble fibers called beta-glucans, which may help with satiety and metabolic health.

Resistant starch may be found in both brown and white rice, especially if it is cooked and then allowed to cool. While white rice is undoubtedly OK, brown rice has extra nutrients, particularly fiber, which may aid in your healthy weight reduction efforts.

Refined grains, such as white bread and the majority of commercial baked goods, are OK as long as they are consumed in moderation and not as the main component of your diet.

Also keep in mind that certain items labeled "whole grain" on the label may be highly processed and, if consumed in excess, may lead to undesirable weight gain.

Chili p.
Consuming chili peppers might be beneficial while trying to lose weight.

They contain capsaicin, which gives hot peppers like chilies their fiery flavor. According to certain research, capsaicin can boost your feeling of fullness and speed up the metabolism of fat in your body. Together, they might help you on your path to a healthy weight reduction. This chemical is even available as a supplement and is a typical component of many popular weight loss products. This is due to research suggesting that supplements containing capsaicin may speed up metabolism.

However, a review research indicated that compared to people who did not take capsaicin supplements, this impact only resulted in an additional 33 calories burnt per day on average. More study is required to understand this impact, particularly as it relates to capsaicin from dietary sources. Additionally, those who were used to consuming spicy food did not have any negative effects, showing that a certain amount of tolerance may develop.

Fruit is generally regarded as wholesome by health professionals.

People who consume the most fruits and vegetables tend to be healthier than those who don't, according to several demographic studies.

The majority of fruits contain qualities that make them excellent for aiding in the attainment or maintenance of a healthy weight. Therefore, there's no need to avoid them on your road to health.

Despite having natural sugar, fruits are low in calorie density and rich in micronutrients. Additionally, the fiber in them slows the rate at which the sugar is released into your system.

Those who are on an extremely low carb diet or who have an intolerance may wish to avoid or limit fruit. The majority of fruits may help you achieve a healthy weight goal while also being delightful complements.

Grapefruit
Fruits like grapefruit, which are rich in nutrients and fiber, can encourage feelings of fullness.

Eating half a fresh grapefruit before meals resulted in a 3.5-pound weight loss in an earlier research from 2006 that followed 91 obese people for 12 weeks (1.6 kg). A metabolic disorder called insulin resistance was also less prevalent in the grapefruit group.

Therefore, consuming half a grapefruit 30 minutes before meals may help you feel fuller and consume less calories overall. You would be better off, though, eating a variety of fruits and vegetables at each meal because this is not a sustainable practice. If you use certain drugs, such as statins or blood pressure meds, stay away from grapefruit and its juice since it can enhance or interfere with their effects.

More studies on humans are still required to fully understand how grapefruit affects weight reduction and weight control.

Chia Seeds
One of the world's most nutrient-dense foods may be chia seeds. Each ounce (28 grams) has 12 grams of carbohydrates, roughly 10 of which are fiber. Chia seeds are low in carbohydrates and, at 35% of their weight in fiber, are one of the greatest sources of fiber available.

The high fiber content in chia seeds causes them to swell and become gel-like in your stomach. In one experiment, 24 individuals were given either 0.33 ounces (7 grams) or 0.5 ounces (14 grams) of chia seeds with yogurt as a mid-morning snack, and those who did so reported feeling more full.

Additionally, the rich omega-3 fatty acid content of chia seeds may help with weight management. Chia seeds may help you achieve a healthy weight because of their nutritious profile

Whole, Full-Fat Greek Yogurt
Another great dairy product is yogurt. Given that Greek yogurt has twice as much protein as normal yogurt, it is particularly beneficial for weight control. Additionally, certain yogurt varieties, such as Greek yogurt, include probiotic bacteria that help enhance the health of your stomach.

To further improve gut health, look for labels that mention "living cultures" or "active cultures." If you don't see them, seek for a combination of probiotic strains in the ingredients list, such as S. thermophilus or Bifidus.

Leptin resistance, one of the primary hormonal causes of obesity, as well as inflammation may be prevented by having a healthy gut.

Choose yogurt with live, active cultures instead of other varieties, which may have little or no probiotics.

Also, think about selecting full-fat yogurt. Although the data is currently conflicting, some studies indicate that full-fat dairy products, but not low-fat dairy, are linked to a decreased risk of obesity and type 2 diabetes over the long term. It's advised to consume flavored or sweetened low-fat yogurt only sometimes and to read the nutrition label if you're trying to avoid such ingredients as they usually include fillers or extra sugars to make up for texture.

Many meals are scrumptious, healthy, and helpful in achieving or maintaining a healthier weight. The majority of them are entire foods, such as fish, lean meat, produce, fruit, nuts, seeds, and legumes.

Oatmeal and probiotic yogurt are two wonderful examples of minimally processed meals.

Eating these nutritious meals ought to assist in paving the path to a healthy life, along with moderation and regular exercise.

CHAPTER SEVEN

HOW TO BREAK AN ADDICTION TO EATING.

It might seem hard to lose weight when eating is one of your greatest pleasures and exercising is one of your biggest enemies. But even minor adjustments may have a major impact, and there are methods to adapt your way of life so that you consume less calories, burn more of them, and still feel content.

Plan Ahead

Making a weight reduction plan gives you accountability and supports you when you're struggling. Your strategy should contain both short- and long-term objectives, suggestions for wholesome meals and snacks, training schedules, sources of encouragement, and suggestions for lifestyle modifications you might use to lose weight. It's crucial that your plan includes techniques you really believe in and can adhere to for a lifetime, not just momentarily if you want to maintain the weight you lose.

Shift It!

Even though increasing your regular physical activity won't result in weight loss on its own, it will help you manage your weight. Dietary changes rather than exercise are more helpful for losing weight, according to dietician at the Mayo Clinic, but even just 30 minutes a day of walking can add another 1/3 pound to your weekly weight reduction. You're likely to lose weight even more quickly if you discover a sport or exercise you enjoy and wish to partake in frequently. An hour of basketball, football, or tennis burns more than 700 calories for a 200-pound person!

Eat Up!
Cutting calories doesn't need you to constantly be hungry or consume salad for every meal. If you enjoy eating, then indulge, but make sure that the majority of your diet consists of wholesome, low-calorie meals. Are you prone to binge on fatty treats like pie, cake, chips, and other things? Consume similar foods that are healthier. For instance, swap out an ice cream bar for a frozen banana, a baked spiced apple for apple pie, and packaged potato chips for baked vegetable chips. If you do indulge, only consume a modest portion. If you choose to drink water instead of soda or juice, you'll also save a lot of extra calories.

Reorganize Your Portions
If you alter the portions of each food type you eat, you may have a full plate of food at each meal and still lose weight. According to the USDA, you should put 50 percent of your plate toward fruits and vegetables, 25 percent toward whole grains, and 25 percent toward items high in protein, such as stir-

fried tofu or lean turkey breast. A tiny serving of dairies, such as a glass of nonfat milk or a piece of low-fat string cheese, can be served on the side.

Considerations

Consult with your doctor or a certified dietitian if the idea of coming up with nutritious food ideas intimidates you or if you're unsure of where to start when creating a weight reduction strategy. If you need assistance creating a plan you can stick to, track your development over time, and schedule a follow-up appointment if you don't notice progress within six to eight weeks.

How Long Will It Take Me to Get Fit?

Being "ripped" takes far longer than six weeks, despite some commercials' claims of dramatic fitness improvements, It is impossible to accurately estimate how long it will take to become in shape.

It takes different amounts of time to reach different goals, such as strength, endurance, weight loss, body fat reduction, etc.

Increasing your amount of physical exercise will likely improve your mood before you notice any changes. The sort of exercise used and a person's starting fitness level are crucial factors. Although some advertising may lead you to believe differently, becoming healthy is not simple. Even "natural" exercisers won't see immediate improvements in fitness. A previous investigation from the University of Wisconsin, examined whether or not six weeks of training would significantly enhance fitness and beauty. The results were published in The Journal of Strength and Conditioning Research in 2004.

The researchers gave 25 sedentary guys a 6-week fitness program that included three 20-minute aerobic sessions each week or three 30-minute bouts of high-intensity, total-body strength training. At the start and end of the study, a group of specialists rated the men's appearances based on pictures. After six weeks, the ratings remained steady. The men's perceptions of their own attractiveness remained mostly unaltered after six weeks. In addition, objective fitness measures including body fat percentage, the number of pushups performed, and oxygen efficiency did not rise during the course of the study.

If six weeks is not enough time to get in shape, how long does it take?
Depending on the goals, time

The answer to this fitness question depends in part on how you define "in shape." Your time frame for reaching your fitness goals may vary.
A novice will need less time to become in shape for a 5K race than they will to train for their first triathlon or marathon. They will also need a different training

program than someone getting ready for a week-long camping excursion.

You might not feel as out of breath as you do when you run to catch the train or climb the stairs. Or having the stamina to play outside without getting tired with your grandchildren.

If you don't yet have a "ripped physique," you shouldn't disregard these small changes, the mental advantages of exercising are much more essential than the visible improvements we are all so keen to see.

This includes more drive and assurance to continue exercising till you begin to experience bodily advantages. Additionally, you will soon experience even larger fitness benefits if you exercise consistently. Your fitness and health may undergo a substantial transformation in three to four months. You can plainly see some changes after 6 to 8 weeks, with each strength taking about the same amount of time.

"Three months is typically a suitable time limit for a customer who is already in great heart condition but merely wants to learn how to lift weights properly, when will you thus begin to have a "ripped body"?

if you maintain a balanced diet and exercise program for a full year and you weren't overly overweight to begin with, you should be able to see your six-pack.

Getting into shape to compete
Not everyone enjoys exercising only for the sake of exercising. There are several outdoor races to select from, including 5K or 10K running events, marathons, half-marathons, and 100-mile cycling rides, for those who need a target to keep motivated.

For those who enjoy variety, there are also triathlons, Tough Mudders, Super Spartans, and other obstacle events.

It is even more crucial to take your time getting in shape if you have a really specific fitness goal. "If you are training for an event or race, please be over-prepared," said a certified personal trainer from Primal Power in New York.

Three to four months before to an endurance event like the Spartan race, you should start jogging five miles if you have never done it before. Despite the fact that our bodies get stronger, you want to sprint rather than stomp to the finish line.

You may use a variety of training plans to get in shape for these events, but you should plan to dedicate at least two months to pre-race preparation, clocking miles 3–6 days per week.

Even for novices, the extra time will be worthwhile.

In a 2007 study published in the European Journal of Applied Physiology, researchers prepared an untrained group of people for a half- and full-marathon over the course of nine months. People who participated in the program boosted their VO2 max by 24% by the conclusion of the research.

Expect to put in significant mileage to be in shape, even if you favor noncompetitive outdoor pursuits like camping, kayaking, or mountain biking.

These are two days that are back-to-back, full eight-hour days with a loaded pack. Despite the fact that it can appear challenging, many newbies have previously taken it this way. Silberberg thinks that many people may go on a hiking trip immediately. The second day is the toughest since your enthusiasm has faded and you already have sore feet and muscles from the first day.

fitness-related factors
Of all, these are only basic recommendations.

Your journey might be sped up or slowed down by various factors along the route.

How fit you are when you start is one factor that, in my experience, influences each person's unique success timetable.

Your choice of exercise is crucial and will affect you differently depending on whether you are a beginner or are recuperating from an illness or accident. if you're new to exercise or maybe you're being cautious because of an injury, the results of walking for 90 minutes a day would be different from those of someone who is used to exercise and has decided to engage in a HIIT program.

However, because they are starting lower on the fitness scale and need less activity to challenge their bodies, beginners may advance more quickly.

With appropriate training, beginners "experience significant gains in strength across the board every week."

Naturally, your exercise program's input has an impact on the outcomes as well. According to Kingsford, if you only feel like exercising at a level 6 on a scale of 1 to 10, you won't see the same results as someone who feels like exercising at a level 9.

Researchers separated sedentary, overweight, or obese women into three groups and had them exercise at levels of 50, 100, or 150 percent of the advised energy expenditure in a study.

After six months, women who exercised with the highest intensity experienced an 8% increase in their cardiovascular fitness. The lowest intensity group experienced a 4% improvement in fitness. If you've been inactive for a while, an 8 percent boost in fitness may not seem like much, but it may make a significant difference.

If you up the intensity even further, the results will happen faster. However, you won't notice any benefits if you don't work hard enough. Strike a balance and understand that being healthy and active has nothing to do with competition or achievement.

putting on weight
If your workout practice becomes engrained in your schedule, you'll probably find it's easier to maintain. However, an accident, illness, or just the demands of daily life can swiftly put a stop to your workouts.

According to a performance coach and trainer, "Life challenges will always knock you off your plan at some time, but the most important thing is to return back to your program and persist in it for the long term." Cardiovascular fitness often suffers first.

If you're well trained and decide to quit working out, your cardio will decrease first and fastest. According to a trained strength and conditioning consultant and top trainer at Exercise.com, who talked with Health line, it will drastically decrease after just a few weeks of inactivity.

According to the American College of Sports Medicine (ACSM), physiological changes, such as those in blood lipoproteins or the body's ability to use glucose for energy, may occur one to two weeks after you stop exercising.

A 1984 Study
Additionally, it was shown by Respiratory, a Reliable Source in the Journal of Applied Physiology Environmental and Exercise Physiology, that endurance athletes' VO2 max reduced by 7% during the first 21 days of inactivity.

This stabilized after 56 days of no exercise. The athletes' VO2 max was greater than that of non-athletes even after 84 days of inactivity.

Muscle power could last longer during a break.
According to a study from 2000, young individuals only lost 8% of their strength after 31 weeks of inactivity, according to Trusted Source in Medicine and Science in Sports and Exercise. Older people lost 14% of their power over that time.

Between 12 and 31 weeks, the strength decreased most significantly. Even short breaks could not have an influence on your overall strength gain.

According to a 2011 study that appeared in the journal Trusted Source in Clinical Physiology and Functional Imaging, rookie bench pressers who took a 3-week break in the middle of a 15-week program had the same results as those who stuck with it.

As a result, if your foundation is solid, it stays with you.

Resistance training permanently changes the physiology of your muscle cells, even after a long break from exercise.

This quickens the process of regaining strength and development after a significant break from the gym. For overall fitness, the same holds true.

The effects of a break from exercise can vary from person to person.

But the longer and more often you've been working out and training, the less of an impact a break will have on you.

The good news is that you can prevent fitness losses over a break by exercising consistently, even if it's at a lesser level than before. According to the ACSM, all you need to do to keep up your current level of strength, performance, and health advantages is one session per week of moderate- to hard-intensity exercise. What you do to get through a break will depend on the circumstances.

If life got in the way and you stopped working out, you might need to squeeze in physical exercise whenever you can. For instance, you could have to ride a bike to work or do bodyweight resistance exercises all day.

If you are injured, you may need to significantly modify your workout regimen. I urge students who have been hurt to continue going to the gym and exercising, but we absolutely alter their program to accommodate the injured body part, depending on the severity of the injury. For example, a student with a shoulder problem can still come and work out their lower body to prevent being completely deconditioned.

It's essential to work with a doctor or physical therapist to develop a regimen that will keep you active while also enabling your body to heal.

As an injured joint heals, people "need to learn to trust the afflicted joint again. Favoring the unaffected side once therapy ends just increases the risk of sustaining another injury elsewhere in the body. After a protracted time of inactivity, it is often preferable to restart, working with your current level of health and fitness rather than where you were before the break.

For it, you'll need a lot of the same patience that got you in shape in the first place. Yes, depending on your background. According to a certified personal trainer with the New York City-based Primal Power, "when working on a short-term purpose of getting in shape," "you have to know your starting location and your prior experience."

If you are a beginner, weekend warrior, or experienced competitor, different training programs will work better for you. Similar to how "fit" you may get in a month.

Couch-To-Fit Program For 30 Days
If you are new to working out or have recently returned from a long vacation, I suggest starting with a cardiovascular regimen.

Jog or run for 20 to 30 minutes every other day. You can also do moderate-intensity activities like brisk walking, swimming, and biking. After your cardiovascular workout, do three to four rounds of bodyweight exercises like squats, pushups, lunges, burpees, or Russian twists.

You'll need to rest for a day after these workouts, but I suggest continuing your exercise by studying yoga to reduce stress, increase blood flow, and increase flexibility. After that, progressively add strength training. You'll experience an increase in metabolism, which will help you burn more calories and fat. If you have access to a gym, I also advise completing three to four sets of strength exercises with 12 to 16 repetitions per session. Exercises like leg presses, rows, lat pulldowns, and chest presses may be included in this. A personal trainer may help you develop a home strength program using bodyweight exercises, dumbbells, and kettlebells if there isn't a gym nearby.

Exercise with short bursts of intensity

Full-body strengthening workouts and high-intensity interval training are suggested by Marks for quick results.

Sculpting your muscles and burning fat are two goals that may be achieved at once with this sort of program. In high-intensity interval training, periods of severe activity are interspersed with periods of moderate exercise or rest. Even with shorter exercises, this can still have positive outcomes. I will advise setting a goal of engaging in high-intensity interval training three days a week with one day off in between.

Exercise for 30 to 60 seconds at a moderate intensity, followed by 30 to 60 seconds at a strong intensity. For 20 to 30 minutes, repeat this cycle. This kind of exercise may be carried out on a treadmill, I advise performing 15 to 25 minutes of one-minute "all-out" sprints, followed by two minutes of walking.

If you don't have access to a treadmill, you may instead perform high-knee runs or burpee intervals. Athletes of various skill levels utilize high-intensity interval training to increase their fitness. Even novices may use it with some adjustment. You may conduct very hard power walking by swinging your arms rather than holding onto the treadmill and following the same interval pattern if you are not a runner or are just starting your exercise regimen.

Increase the treadmill inclination or walking pace for the cycle's intense portion.

This exercise can also be performed outside on a track or sidewalk with steps or hills acting as the slope. Circuit training, a quick-paced combination of cardio and weights, is another quick yet intensive workout.

The shortening of the rest period is the main component of circuit training. Performance improves with increased repetition volume and shorter rest periods.

Increasing your game
If you currently engage in regular exercise, you might choose to pick one goal for the month.

A certified personal trainer advises focusing on "a specific performance barrier that you haven't quite been able to break through, and setting a clear, quantifiable target."

This may include bench pressing 10 pounds heavier than normal or speeding up your two-mile run by two minutes. Restructure your training plan once you've chosen a target for the month to help you achieve it.

You will become much more concentrated when exercising as a result, and you could discover that your commitment to your workout regimen has been renewed. This is because you will have your eyes set on a certain objective that must be achieved within a predetermined time frame.

Advanced weightlifters and athletes who have been consistent for four or five years "will not notice great strength increases within a month, Instead, concentrate on your training volume rather than the intensity of the weight you're moving. actions that increase authority can also be advantageous for this group. Instead of doing the typical cardio exercises like running or riding a bike, consider boxing.

Plyometric exercises, like box jumps and plyo pushups, can also be incorporated into your training routine. Alternately, include additional power workouts like flipping heavy tires or using a push sled or prowler.

setting sensible objectives
Being honest with yourself about what you can do is the greatest method to attain results in a month.

Setting a goal in terms of weight rather than fitness, such as "I will lose 5 pounds before Memorial Day," is one error novices make. This may go awry.

In spite of being in far better shape than when they started, novices sometimes struggle to maintain their weight despite committing to a regular training schedule for a whole month. For beginners, the ability to gain muscle while shedding fat is fairly common.

This "failure" can make people give up exercising when the month is through.

Beginners can set unrealistic goals for themselves, such as wanting to lose 20 pounds and get six-pack abs in a month, from their exercises.

I advise newcomers to pay more attention to their conduct at the beginning than their physical outcomes. Consider stating your objective as "I will aim to do four exercises each week for the next month," rather than "I will lose 5 pounds in 30 days."

By changing the focus in this way, the objective becomes more reachable; the only way to fail is to give up completely. It also lessens some of the pressure to perform flawlessly.

Because most beginning exercisers haven't yet formed the exercise habit, "I particularly enjoy these sorts of objectives for beginners because creating the habit is the first step to attaining the kind of long-term fitness outcomes that most people actually want." Better ways to eat and live

Fitness professionals concur that your level of fitness and performance is significantly influenced by the nourishment you put into your body.

eating well on its own may "radically modify an individual's body fat percentage and retain lean body composition."

This entails avoiding processed and quick foods, increasing your intake of fresh foods, particularly fruits and vegetables, and establishing a nutritional balance. Simply reducing your intake of soda, sugar, and alcohol can flatten your stomach.

She also advises that you should attempt to consume calories that are composed of 60% carbs, 20% proteins, and 20% fats. Likewise, drink a lot of water. The more water, the better. Staying well-hydrated will improve the appearance of your skin, reduce your appetite, and even improve your flexibility since it keeps your muscles and ligaments supple, Putting the "fast" back into breakfast by skipping dinner and waiting till morning may even be beneficial.

You will give your body a chance to reset each night by finishing your meal by 7 o'clock, and you'll wake up with a thinner tummy. Eliminating needless late-night munching in front of the TV is one of the perks. However, going to bed sooner will result in having supper earlier.

The optimum time to sleep each night is when it is dark, so try to get to bed around 10 p.m. and wake up at 6 a.m. with the sun.

There is no better time to start than right now, whether you want to reduce weight, grow stronger, or improve your performance over the course of the upcoming month.

The thirty days will fly by, but if you stay on task, you may accomplish a lot. While it is physically impossible to go from being overweight and out of shape to look like a Men's Health cover model by Memorial Day, it is acceptable to expect one month to pass before seeing noticeable improvements in fitness.

CHAPTER EIGHT

The Most Common Fitness Myths.

Discover the reality behind 10 prevalent fitness and workout misconceptions so you can debunk the urban legends.

Many of us receive guidance regarding purported "facts" relating to fitness and exercise from friends, coworkers, and gym pals. The dangers of receiving too little or too much physical exercise are frequently discussed in the news. The majority of those media reports and bits of advice are false, so you shouldn't let them discourage you from working out. In light of this, we made the decision to investigate some of the most well-known fitness misconceptions in further detail. Even the most seasoned athletes can become highly confused by all the information on fitness dos and don'ts, whether it be concerned about joint and body health or not understanding which workout styles are ideal for your specific goals. But don't worry—we have gathered some of the most widespread myths so you can locate the information that will be most useful to you.

"No Gain Without Pain"
Let's start by getting this straight: if you are two-thirds of the way through a spin class or even five minutes into a mountain climb and it feels unpleasant and difficult, that is probably to be anticipated. However, it is definitely a really good idea to stop and consult a physio if you get a sharp ache in your right knee whenever you run or cycle.

While going too easy in the gym won't get you the results you want, going too hard can be detrimental. While going too lightly at the gym won't get you the results you want, going too hard might be detrimental. Finding something difficult is not the same as actually hurting due to an injury. Recognize the burn you experience during exercise and the effort your body is making; if one of these things is happening, stop immediately. Something is amiss if the pain is strong, strange, stinging, or sharp and not what you would typically anticipate with the heat your muscles experience after an exercise. You must deal with the issue.

If you want to lose weight, weight training is not a good idea.
Even though so many individuals have a propensity to avoid the weights section of the gym, here is actually where you need to go if you want to lose weight. A tailored weightlifting exercise with modest weights and high repetitions will tone muscles and burn more calories than an aerobic workout.

The crucial factor is how many calories you burn after your workout. That-after burn for women might contribute up to 350 more calories. And keep in mind that increased muscle mass can also increase the body's metabolic activity, leading to more effective calorie and fat burning overall. Happy days! Your body burns fatter when you consume more protein. You won't turn into the Hulk any time soon from rapid muscle growth, but you will lose weight far more quickly than with just cardio.

Keep Your Aerobic Exercise Intensity Low to Burn More Fat

Let's remove this misconception once and for all since the facts show that although exercise at a low level mostly burns fat, exercise at a high intensity primarily burns carbohydrates. (Since there is a continuum between the two, as activity becomes tougher, more carbohydrates are consumed while less fat is consumed.) The problem is that although harder workouts burn a lot of calories, low-intensity exercise doesn't.

Imagine it like two slices of pie. Due to the low-calorie expenditure, the low-intensity pie contains largely fat storage but very little else. Only a small portion of the calories in the high-intensity pie is derived from fat storage, but—and this is important—the pie is considerably larger since a ton more calories are burned. Making the high-intensity slice is therefore preferable because of its high calorie and hence fat-burning output. Okay?!

Although it is beneficial to burn fat, as you would assume that the only way to lose weight is to burn more calories than you consume, burning more calories is really more crucial for weight loss than burning fat. Don't let the prospect of losing weight generally and advancing your fitness prevent you from engaging in high-intensity, anaerobic exercise.

Step lessons or using a step machine will leave you a big behind.

Stepping is an aerobic, low-resistance exercise unless you've gone completely nuts and increased the stepper's resistance to the point where you can hardly move the pedals. Since it won't provide enough stimulation for muscle tissue to grow as a consequence, it won't have any impact on how big your behind is Stepping is a fantastic cardio exercise that will increase your cardiovascular fitness and increase your muscle endurance in your legs and glutes.

Stepping is a fantastic cardio exercise that will increase your cardiovascular fitness and increase your muscle endurance in your legs and glutes. However, the most important thing to keep in mind is to maintain proper posture. Keep the tailbone slightly tucked under and the navel softly brought to the spine since stepping with your belly out and your back arched will undoubtedly give the illusion of a giant behind! Furthermore, even if an anaerobic activity, the majority of glute workouts won't even result in an enlarged behind. Instead of increasing the behind, working out will cause it to become perkier and more peachy. Large bottoms are caused by extra fat accumulations under the glutes and around the hips, thus toning those muscles and losing that fat can really reshape your behind.

If you walk 10,000 steps a day, you don't need to do any more exercise.
This is a difficult one, I see. It genuinely depends on your objectives. Instead of promoting increased fitness, the 10,000-step recommendation is intended to avoid sickness in those who don't exercise and have grown too used to our automated culture.

Achieving that goal consistently would undoubtedly enhance your fitness if you begin from a sedentary foundation, but it still only counts as low-intensity aerobic exercise. This national goal was created to encourage individuals to include movement in their hectic lives, not to substitute exercise.

Complementing this with shorter, higher-intensity aerobic activity (such as running, participating in a spinning class, or conducting circuit training), strength training (using weights or your own body weight as resistance), and flexibility exercises is great for overall health. It's never ideal to consistently use the same intensity or kind of exercise because each sort of exercise has unique advantages. To keep your body guessing and protect your mind from reaching a monotonous workout plateau, variety is essential.

The best exercise to flatten the stomach is sitting up.
The "six-pack" or rectus abdominis (RA) muscle on the front of the torso is worked by sit-ups, crunches, curls, or really any activity that involves curling your body forward. Unfortunately, exercising this muscle won't make your stomach flatter and won't give you abs. A strong, corset-like muscular strap that wraps around the waist from back to front is hidden deep behind the six-pack. Few of us ever pay any attention to the transversus abdominis (TA), often known as the core, which is the muscle that flattens the stomach.

Put your thumbs on the sides of your waist, level with your navel, and place your other fingers on your pubic bone to activate your TA (the area beneath your belly button). Now, without elevating your ribs or holding your breath, move the region below your belly button backward (away from the fingers). Once you can "activate your core" (as we say in the profession!) practice this frequently throughout the day. There are many more core exercises to strengthen your midsection and flatten your tummy.

"The more water you consume while exercising, the better."
While it is true that we require more fluids when we are exercising, you don't need to drink buckets of

water to keep hydrated. The "glug" method is really counterproductive since the body can only hold so much liquid at once; if you pour in too much, you'll just pee it out again!

Additionally, if you've ever swallowed a bottle of water while jogging, it will seem as though a washing machine has been installed in place of your stomach. Water should replenish the fluids lost during activity, thus ingesting an excessive amount will be useless or even harmful.

Indeed, in extreme circumstances (like lengthy endurance races), you can even put yourself in danger of hyponatremia, a disease that might be deadly. The ideal strategy is to stay well-hydrated all the time, not just before your activity. You won't start off dehydrated if you make sure to consume water and other liquids throughout the day; you can get by just fine consuming a few sips while working out.

And you won't experience uncomfortable stomach slosh! Due to the rise in hyponatremia occurrences in recent years, international sports authorities no longer advise a certain amount of fluid to be consumed during exercise. They now advise drinking when you're thirsty or weighing yourself before and after a timed workout and converting any weight loss in grams to fluid loss in millimeters(For instance, you should strive to drink 500ml of water during subsequent one-hour runs if your running for an hour results in a half-kilogram loss in body weight.)

"Running Hurts Your Knees"
Running has a reputation for damaging knees, but if you train wisely, use the correct running shoes, warm up properly, pay attention to nagging aches, and run on different surfaces, it's actually pretty beneficial for your knees. Running can prevent osteoarthritis by keeping joints and connective tissue strong, flexible, and nourished, according to research in the journal Arthritis and Rheumatism. Running does not increase the risk of joint disorders. Jogging can aggravate shin splints, which are common and can be painful. However, you should only stop running if your shoes are very deficient. While both groups of people suffered some degradation with aging in their knee and hip joints, different research in the Journal of Rheumatology revealed no differences in the degree or pace of degeneration in either group. Therefore, if you have bad knees, don't be deterred from going for a run because it won't be harmful. Just make sure you're prepared for running by stretching and dressing appropriately.

The better it is for you to exercise more.
There might be too much physical activity., believe it or not. You can never reach your full potential if you deny yourself the rest you need since it is during rest, not exercise, that the body does all of the essential repairs and "housekeeping" to make itself fitter and stronger. This isn't an excuse to simply work out once a week and say your body needs a break; that would be stretching it.

While you can do aerobic exercise and flexibility exercises every day, it's wise to follow the "hard, easy" rule, where you follow strenuous training sessions with a gentler workout the following day. This gives your muscles at least 48 hours to recover between strength training workouts of specific body parts.

Additionally, overtraining can weaken your immune system and increase your chance of injury, which may force you to miss several weeks of workouts while you recuperate. When paired with obligations and job, training too hard and for too long may drain your physical and mental vitality. As a result, athletes and individuals burn out much too frequently. Don't worry too much; rest days are an essential component of training, and taking one day off won't hinder your development.

Exercise shouldn't be done too late at night since it will keep you awake.

We've been told for a very long time that only mild exercise, like yoga or Pilates, is appropriate for the later hours of the day. We are told that if we engage in any other form of activity in the evening, we may spend hours laying in bed, awake. Not at all, says a University of California sleep specialist. He discovered that exercising might assist insomniacs fall asleep just as well as sleeping drugs. He recommends people to do their own experiments to see whether exercise improves sleep. Additionally, he discovered that outdoor exercise was superior than indoor exercise for treating sleep issues.

You will become exhausted after working out, and while you often feel terrific afterward, a shower and snooze are a pleasant follow-up. Due to hectic schedules, evening exercises are occasionally the only time of day to squeeze one in. Unlike morning workouts, which can be excellent for boosting metabolism and freeing up the day, evening workouts won't keep you up till the wee hours of the morning.